HOMEOPATHY

FOR BEGINNERS

by
Nica Michelle

Copyright 2017

(Previously published as Homeopathy Hints: For Beginners)

Table of Contents

INTRODUCTION

I was incredibly skeptical about homeopathy at first. In fact, I almost threw my first remedies away without using them. I'm so glad I didn't, because homeopathy has been wonderfully beneficial to my friends and family over the years. It has saved us thousands of dollars and given us peace of mind, because we have the ability to treat ourselves naturally.

Looking back, I see why I was so skeptical; there wasn't a lot of information about homeopathy back then, and what was available was often too detailed for a beginner. This book is for those who want to learn the basics with a short and simple guide that can be read in one sitting.

Homeopathy For Beginners is a compilation of the things I've learned while working with professional homeopaths, attending school, doing research, and through my own trial and error. It represents years of experience and hours of study during my own family's health journey. I hope it gives you the confidence you need to begin using homeopathy.

WHAT IS HOMEOPATHY?

Homeopathy was discovered by Samuel Hahnemann in 1796. It was based on the principle of *like cures like*. This theory suggests that if you find a substance that causes the same symptoms that you're experiencing, you can put that substance in water, dilute it and shake it, and use that dilution or remedy to help with your ailment. Homeopathic remedies are often made out of plants, minerals, or animals; but almost anything can be used to make a remedy. For example, the remedy *rhus toxicodendron* is made from poison ivy. If you have an itchy rash or swollen stiff joints, symptoms you would get if you were exposed to poison ivy, then *rhus toxicodendron* might be a great remedy for you.

Homeopathy is not the same as naturopathy, herbs, essential oils, or other natural treatments. It is a complete and separate form of natural medicine that can help with many health concerns. Many people who use homeopathy believe it has the ability to address the root cause of issues, and that it's one of the safest forms of self care. It directs your body to heal whatever symptoms you are experiencing, instead of acting upon or altering your body like medications or herbs. This is why many people are comfortable using homeopathy on newborn babies, pregnant and nursing moms, and the elderly. Personally, I like homeopathy over other natural treatments, because there is little to no risk for beginners when they follow a few simple rules. As long as you keep these things in mind, you can use homeopathy with confidence:

- Use a resource to match your unique symptoms to a particular remedy.

- Start with the lowest potency and work up to higher potencies.

- Never continue to repeat a remedy that is not working for you.

- Only redose when your symptoms return.

CHOOSING A REMEDY

When you decide you want to address a condition using homeopathy, you'll need to figure out which remedy to use. This can be challenging at first, because homeopathy works much differently than the medicine most people are accustomed to. Most medication and herbs work by treating or suppressing symptoms, instead of addressing the root cause. Homeopathy works by directing your body to fix itself, and only works if you choose a remedy that has been shown to match your unique symptoms.

Let's take a look at an example: the common cold. You won't find one remedy that works for every case of the common cold, because everyone's cold is different. Some people may get a runny nose, while others might get a stuffy nose and a sore throat. Some people may feel their cold more in their chest, but others get a lot of pressure in their sinuses. The different symptoms I've described here match different remedies. One remedy may match well to a stuffy nose and a sore throat, but would be useless for a cold with chest congestion or sinus pressure. At first it can be overwhelming, but with a little practice you'll get the hang of it.

Let's try to pick a remedy. You've come down with a case of the common cold. How do you figure out what to take? The first thing you'll want to do is to make a list of your symptoms. Try to be as descriptive as possible. Include things like how you're feeling emotionally, physical symptoms, anything that makes your symptoms better or worse, and even food cravings. You'll be watching for any strange or peculiar symptoms. Your list might look something like this:

- My nose is dripping like a faucet

- I have burning watery mucous

- I feel like I'll never get better

- My eyes are watery

- My body feels cold

Then you'll need to consult a homeopathic resource to match these symptoms to a remedy. There are a number of good books that describe the most common remedies, or you can look on the internet. Personally, my favorite resource is *Homeopathic Self Care* by Robert Ullman. This book is broken down into sections for many of the most common ailments. It covers things like colds, flus, ear infections, sinus infections, headaches, and more. In this book, you would turn to the section for a common cold and consult the table for a remedy matching these symptoms.

If you were to look on the internet for homeopathic remedies for a cold, you would find many sites that have a list of the most common cold remedies. If you perused the list you would find a remedy called *allium cepa*, which matches many of the symptoms you added to your hypothetical list above. This would be the first remedy to try. *Arsenicum album* is also a good match, if *allium cepa* doesn't work.

There are many other remedies for a common cold, but these two match the symptoms we described very well. This would be a good place to begin. I'll talk about how to administer the remedy in the dosing a remedy section of the book.

POTENCIES

Potency refers to the strength or intensity of a remedy, and is identified by roman numerals. The lowest potency remedies are labeled with an X (e.g. 3X, 6X, 30X). The higher potency remedies are, in order, C, M, CM, and MM.

Different potencies affect the body in different ways. Some people are sensitive to homeopathy, and only need the lower X or C potencies. Others do better with higher potencies in the M range. A homeopath might recommend higher or lower potencies, but if you're on your own you'll want to start with a 30C or 200C.

6C, 30C, and 200C are the most commonly available potencies, and you will often find them in your health food store. Most stores carry remedies made by a company called Boiron. They are packaged in blue or purple hard plastic tubes that cost about six to eight dollars.

It's important to note that a lower potency remedy does not need to match your symptoms as closely as a higher potency remedy. If you're not sure if you have the right remedy, it's best to pick a lower potency.

DOSING A REMEDY

Dosing homeopathy is quite different than dosing traditional medication or herbs. The number of pills taken at once doesn't really matter. You can think of homeopathic remedies as a map for your body. Let's say your friend asks you for directions to your house. You could print out one map or multiple copies of the same map and give them to her. No matter what, she would find her way to your house, but the extra copies of the map don't help her get there any faster. It's the same with remedies; any number of remedy pills will direct your body to fix the issue you're addressing. If you take one pill or ten pills at a time, the result is the same. You really only need one, but if the pills are smaller, I like to take two or three to make sure I'm getting a good dose.

The important thing to remember is that homeopathic dosing is based on potency and frequency, not the number of pills. You may need to repeat a dose every fifteen minutes, sometimes you'll need it once an hour, other times once a week, and sometimes one dose is enough and your symptoms won't return. It depends on the remedy, your overall health, and the issue you're trying to improve.

Homeopathy can be dosed a number of ways. The most common delivery mechanism is a dose on a sugar pellet, which can be either lactose or sucrose. This is called a "dry dose" and the pellets are what you find in the remedy bottles you purchase at the store or homeopathic pharmacy. Dosing with these is simple and works well for most people. Another way to dose is to put the dry pellet in a small amount of water and let it dissolve. Then drink or take sips from the water. This is commonly called a "water dose" and seems to be a gentler way to take remedies. If you are especially sensitive, you can dissolve a lower potency remedy in a cup of water and then give a drop of that water. This tends to have a milder effect than dry dosing or water dosing.

Like I mentioned above, if you're beginning homeopathy on your own, you should probably start with a lower potency like a 30C. Once you have the remedy in hand that best matches your symptoms, pour one large pellet or two smaller pellets into the lid of the bottle. Drop the remedy directly under your tongue and let it dissolve. If you accidentally chew it or move it around in your mouth, don't worry! It will still work. Wait for fifteen to thirty minutes (remember, everyone responds differently) and check your symptom list to see if your symptoms have had any noticeable improvements.

Let's say you notice you're feeling better. This means you're on the right track! Now, the best thing to do is wait until your symptoms worsen or you develop new symptoms. If your symptoms get better but come back, dose the same remedy again. If your symptoms evolve, it means you may have moved into the next stage of your illness and it's time to find a new remedy. Pick a different remedy using the steps outlined in my "Choosing a Remedy" section.

If the remedy didn't help at all, try it once or twice more. Remember to wait fifteen to thirty minutes between each dose. If you still don't notice a difference, pick a different remedy using the steps in "Choosing a Remedy." Sometimes you have to try two or three remedies before you find the right one. Just keep trying.

It's important to remember that you should **NEVER** continue taking a remedy if it doesn't produce a noticeable improvement in your symptoms. Pay attention to this, because continuing to take a remedy you don't need will eventually cause your body to start exhibiting the symptoms that remedy matches. This is often referred to as proving a remedy. Proving occurs when you take a remedy that you don't need more than two or three times, or when you take a remedy you do need, but too often.

Let's get back to the common cold example: You take a dose of *allium cepa* every twenty minutes for an hour and each time it's really helping you to feel better. Your nose quits running so much, your eyes stop watering, and you don't feel as chilly. Then you notice some different symptoms occurring, and *allium cepa* isn't helping anymore. It's time to change remedies. Write a new list of symptoms and proceed to match them to a new remedy. Because homeopathy encourages your body heal itself, you often will see your symptoms change as your body works to fix the issue. This is normal, and an important part of the healing process.

WATER DOSING

Water plays a big part in the process of making homeopathic remedies, and it can play a big part in dosing them as well. If you are especially sensitive to remedies, you can dissolve a lower potency remedy in a cup of water. Then stir and drink the water, or take one drop from it for an even gentler effect.

You can also use water to conserve remedy pellets. If you are running low on a remedy, or just want to conserve, you can put a few pellets in a plastic water bottle. Let them dissolve, and then shake the bottle up really well. From there you can take a sip from the bottle whenever you need a dose of the remedy. One sip is equivalent to one dose. Make sure you shake the bottle between doses. You'll want to store the bottle in the refrigerator, it will only last a few days and then you'll need to remake it. In my experience, remedies prepared this way work fairly well, but the effects don't last quite as long. It may be different for you, but it's a good idea to experiment with water dosing to see how it works.

WHAT SHOULD I EXPECT TO SEE

How do you know if you picked the correct remedy? This is one of the most commonly asked questions about homeopathy, and can be answered with just one word: change. Change might look like a better attitude toward life or an overall feeling of well-being. You could also see a change in your physical symptoms or a combination of all of these. It can look like a lot of different things, but the correct remedy will always yield results. You might notice a dramatic change in your symptoms right away, or it might be more subtle. If that sounds vague to you, it's because results vary from person to person. As you use homeopathy, you'll get a feel for how your body responds to remedies.

If you try a remedy for an acute condition and you don't notice a change after fifteen to thirty minutes, try another dose. If you still don't see positive change after another fifteen to thirty minutes, you most likely chose the incorrect remedy. Go back to the list of possible remedies and try the next best option.

Occasionally, you may notice a negative impact from taking a remedy. This is usually pretty rare, but if you experience negative effects from a remedy, there could be a few reasons. You may have chosen the correct remedy, but the potency you used was incorrect. You also may have chosen a remedy that is a very close match for you, but not quite right. If you experience either of these, you can either wait until the remedy wears off, or if the symptoms are too uncomfortable, consider trying a zapper. I discuss zappers in the next section.

WHAT IF SOMETHING GOES WRONG

It is possible to take too much of a remedy; either dosing too frequently or taking a higher potency than what is needed. If this happens, it can cause your symptoms to worsen noticeably before getting better. This is commonly referred to as an aggravation. If you find that you are aggravating on a remedy, you may want to try using a lower potency next time. Usually I try to wait it out, but if this happens to you and you really aren't feeling well, you can make a zapper.

To make a zapper, put a pellet of the remedy you need to zap into a glass of water. Let it dissolve and stir it up. Then dump and fill the cup of water ten to fifteen times in a row. Now, you have a zapper for that remedy. Take a spoon full of that water, and it should help you to feel better in a few minutes. If the symptoms start to return after taking the zapper, dump and rinse the cup two to three more times and take another spoonful. I've used this several times and, though it seems strange, it really helps.

There may be times when you wish to completely stop the action or antidote a remedy. You should only need to do this in the rarest of circumstances; when you are having an adverse reaction to a remedy. Antidoting involves taking another substance or remedy that stops the effect of the currently acting remedy.

Some remedies can be antidoted with strong smelling substances. A good example of this is the essential oil peppermint. Smelling peppermint essential oil will often stop the effects of a remedy. However, more often than not, you will need to look online for a list of remedies that are known to antidote your active remedy. The remedy *camphora* is a common antidote for many other remedies. If you are unable to find an antidote for the remedy you wish to stop, *camphora* is a good one to try. Should you find yourself taking two remedies concurrently, it's important to remember that remedies can antidote each other.

WHERE TO ACQUIRE REMEDIES

There are many ways to acquire homeopathic remedies. The most convenient place to get them is your local health food store. Unfortunately, their selection of remedies can be limited. The bottles often cost around eight dollars each and only contain a small amount of large pellets. In my experience, the best way to purchase remedies is from a homeopathic pharmacy. Buying from a pharmacy has its pitfalls as well: you have to wait to receive your remedy by mail, and many pharmacies are starting to require that you work with a homeopath before they will sell to you. However, there are some that don't. I'll list a few of my favorite homeopathic pharmacies later in this book.

When you purchase from a pharmacy you can get a larger bottle filled with more pellets, and more often than not you can choose the size of the pellets. If you order small or medium size pellets the number of doses in a bottle can dramatically increase, which makes the bottles stretch farther and saves you money!

COMBINATION REMEDIES

Many people are introduced to homeopathy through a combination remedy. You can find them in health food stores, and even some of the large chain stores are selling them now. Combination remedies are made by taking multiple remedies designed to address a specific ailment and applying them to a single pellet. This eliminates the need to match your symptoms to a remedy. There are combos for the common cold, flu, seasonal allergies, coughs, headaches, and more. At first glance they seem like a great way to begin using homeopathy, and they can be very effective. But, while they will often help, they do have their pitfalls.

A combination remedy can contain two or more remedies; the most common remedies for whatever illness the combo addresses. This really takes the guess work and research out of homeopathy. But, combos only work if your symptoms match one of the remedies in the combo. This can be cause for concern, because you are taking several remedies that you don't need every time you use a combo. This leaves you open to proving the other remedies if you take the combo remedy too much. This may be why manufacturers often use low potencies in their combos: it helps to prevent people from proving the remedies they don't need, and lower potencies can be effective even if your symptoms don't match the remedy exactly. Unfortunately, you may need higher potencies to see significant improvement when you don't feel well. Additionally, a combo will only work for you if the remedy you need is in the combo. If it's not in the combo, the combo may not work. I worry this often causes people to abandon homeopathy because they tried a combo and it didn't help, so they assumed homeopathy doesn't work for them.

But, combos do have their uses. Sometimes, the combos can contain remedies that are harder to find locally. Once I had a horrible cough and matched the remedy *coccus cacti* exactly. I didn't have that remedy, and it's not very common, so I couldn't find it locally. Then I got the idea to look for it in a combination remedy. I found it in a low potency combination cough syrup, so I bought it and took it. While it didn't completely cure the cough, it helped enough to where I could get some good sleep and my body took care of the cough on its own.

While combination remedies have a few drawbacks, they definitely have their place, especially when you're a beginner. Just remember that you're taking multiple remedies at once, and try not to overdo it.

CELL SALTS

Cell salts are very low potency homeopathic remedies. They commonly come in larger bottles with puffy quick dissolve tablets, instead of the standard homeopathic pellet. But, they can come on a normal pellet if you order them from a homeopathic pharmacy. They are labeled with numbers, one through twelve, but also have remedy names like *calcarea sulphurica* and *magnesia sulphurica*.

These are general purpose remedies, and are used to help with things like muscle cramps (cell salt #8), indigestion or acid reflux (cell salt #10), or even the sniffles at the start of a cold (cell salt #4). You can find instructions for using them right on the bottle. They are a great way to ease into using homeopathy.

ACUTE VS CHRONIC

When you first start using homeopathy it's best to stick to using remedies for acute, or short-term, issues. Acute issues should be pretty straightforward, and there are often only a handful of remedies to choose from. Using remedies for colds, headaches, flu, and other minor issues will give you good feel for homeopathy, and help to build your confidence in choosing remedies for yourself.

Chronic health issues can be difficult to address, requiring multiple remedies and varying potencies. Homeopathy can help chronic issues like arthritis, chronic fatigue, emotional issues, behavioral issues, autoimmunity, diabetes, eating disorders, asthma, irritable bowel, and more. These cases are best handled by a homeopath that can go over all of your history and suggest the best remedies for you. If you have a complex condition, you should really consult a homeopath.

If your health issues are less complex, you can feel comfortable trying to resolve them on your own first. I've had success finding remedies on my own for things like insomnia, headaches, minor injuries, colds, flus, ear infections, coughs, seasonal allergies, and many others. But, always remember: if you are experiencing a serious health condition or emergency, consult a doctor right away. As always, exercise common sense.

TYPES OF HOMEOPATHY

Once you decide you need a homeopath, either to help with a chronic condition or just to help your family achieve better health, you'll need to decide which homeopath is best for you. You can consult many homeopaths by phone or video chat, so even if you don't have one in your area you still have options available to you. There are many different techniques homeopaths use when choosing remedies. It is important you understand these techniques, so you can decide which would work best for you. I'll highlight a few of the most common methods.

Constitutional homeopathy is one technique, and many homeopaths use it to help with chronic conditions. Constitutional homeopathy involves choosing one remedy that matches an individual as a whole, and giving that remedy to boost the body enough that it can combat its ailment. Many homeopaths who advise this way only give one remedy at a time, and recommend only taking it once a week or less. This method can be effective for some people, and might work well for you if you were particularly healthy before becoming ill.

Adaptational homeopathy is a variation of constitutional homeopathy. An adaptational homeopath is looking for a remedy that matches the individual as a whole. Additionally, the homeopath is also looking for other remedies to support the body; simultaneously addressing acute issues and the individual's predisposition to specific diseases. They may suggest dosing more frequently, and will often have you taking multiple remedies concurrently.

Many homeopaths are becoming certified in a technique called CEASE. CEASE operates on the principle that if constitutional homeopathy isn't working, there must be something happening in the body that is blocking it. CEASE works by clearing out those blocks in the body, so that constitutional remedies can work more effectively. For instance, you may need to clear a chronic bacterial infection or a medication reaction before constitutional homeopathy will work for you. A CEASE homeopath will use special remedies to clear one or more blocks in the body, and then go back to using the constitutional remedy.

Protocol based homeopathy is another method that is becoming more common. Protocol homeopathy uses the same remedies for specific ailments with less consideration of the individual, much like modern medicine will give a medication whenever particular symptoms are present or a diagnoses is given. Anytime an individual has a particular ailment, the same remedy is always given. While this can be effective, and it may be easier to follow a protocol rather than trying to match individual symptoms; it's also much easier to prove a remedy that your body does not need.

I've found I have the best results with homeopaths who use a combination of these styles when suggesting remedies. I like this approach, because I can work with my homeopath to develop a plan that is tailored to my specific needs. Sometimes taking one remedy at a time infrequently is enough, but often my family needs multiple remedies. We've seen the most improvement with this approach.

A few other things to keep in mind: homeopaths have their own areas of expertise. Some of them are general practitioners that have a breadth of experience with many different health issues, while others specialize in specific ailments. If you have a tough case, I would highly recommend finding one that has a lot of experience with the issues you wish to address.

CARING FOR MY REMEDIES

Over the years, I've purchased a lot of remedies. When you've put a lot of money into your remedies you'll want to make sure they are properly protected. The most important things you should avoid exposing your remedies to are heat and sunlight. Don't store them in the bathroom, because heat and steam from the shower can affect your remedies. Depending on your climate, you may want to avoid storing remedies in your car, especially on a hot day. Also, sunlight can deactivate the remedies if they are exposed too much, so keep them out of the sun. Some people suggest that electromagnetic fields can negatively affect your remedies, but I've never experienced that. However, to be safe I do try to keep them away from wall outlets, cell phones, and our wireless router. I currently keep my remedies on a shelf in my closet.

Another thing to keep in mind: homeopathic remedies are made in water and sprayed onto the pellets. This means that it is possible to rub the remedy off of a pellet. You should avoid touching the remedy directly if you can, and just pour the remedy into the lid of the vial and drop it straight into your mouth from the lid. I've yet to have a problem with gently touching a remedy, but I would definitely be careful, and try not create too much friction on the pellet.

It's also not a good idea to reuse vials for different remedies or potencies; the old potencies or remedies might still be in the empty bottle and could cross contaminate any new pills you add to the empty vial. However, it's fine to refill an empty vial with the same remedy and potency it previously contained.

HOMEOPATHIC KITS

Many pharmacies will carry homeopathic kits which contain a variety of common remedies and potencies. There are all kinds of kits: kits that address specific acute issues, child birth, travel, and many others. I recommend using homeopathy for a while to see how you and your family respond to it, and then decide which kit would benefit you the most.

When you've got a good feel for how homeopathy works for you, a kit is a great thing to invest in. While the initial cost up front can seem a bit steep, it is a very cost effective way to acquire a nice collection of remedies. The remedies in most kits end up costing about two dollars per vial, so the kit is an economic way get the remedies you'd want to have on hand. Having a good variety of remedies on hand makes it much easier to use homeopathy when an acute issue arises. My kit has saved me many trips to the doctor when I've had minor issues, and it has paid for itself over and over again.

You could also make your own kit if you can't find one with the remedies you want. You can purchase small essential oil vials online, and then fill them with the homeopathic remedies you use the most. The best storage option I've found for a custom kit is a bullet box from a sporting goods store. Find the box with the correct size compartments for your vials, and you've got a portable storage box for your remedies! I've also used a small zippered coin pouch to store remedies when I can't take my whole kit with me.

BOOK RECOMMENDATIONS

There are a few amazing books out there that are great for the beginner. *Homeopathic Self Care* By Robert Ullman is the book I started out with. It lists many common acute conditions, and the corresponding remedies in a chart format that makes it easy to find a match for your symptoms. The first edition of this book is available for just a few dollars on Amazon, which makes this an affordable option when you are getting started.

Another good option is the book *The Family Guide to Homeopathy* by Dr. Andrew Locke. While it doesn't have the remedies listed in chart format, it does have quality lists of remedies to try for each ailment. It's also a fairly inexpensive way to get started.

Once you get comfortable addressing your acute illnesses with homeopathy, you might consider getting a homeopathic repertory. The repertory is a large book, which lists symptoms and the remedies that match them. You can look up a few of your unusual symptoms, and then cross reference to see if there is a common remedy that will match all of your symptoms. This is how a professional homeopath would help you find remedies for more serious health issues. The repertory can be a difficult book to learn, because you have to be familiar with how it refers to symptoms and determine the section in which to look. It can also be very helpful in finding obscure remedies, especially if you're not able to afford the help of a homeopath at the moment.

PHARMACY RECOMMENDATIONS

You can find many remedies at your local health food store. If you can't find what you need there, you'll need to order online from a pharmacy. The remedies from the store usually come in large pellets, and only have a handful of doses per container. It's much cheaper to buy remedies from a homeopathic pharmacy. Homeopathic pharmacies also carry remedies and potencies that you won't find in a health food store. You can order various sizes of bottles and pellets, which means you can get a lot more of a remedy for the same price.

When you order from a pharmacy, you will need to choose the bottle size, which is measured in drams. A two dram bottle is about the size of a bottle you would find in a health food store, but contains many more pellets. Depending on the pharmacy, you may choose your pellet size. Pharmacies that do this will have a guide to help you choose the pellet size you want on their website. Many pharmacies will only sell to you if you are currently consulting with a homeopath, but

there a few that you can use without seeing
homeopath:

> Washington Homeopathics
> homeopathyworks.com

> Hahnemann Labs
> hahnemannlabs.com

> Helios
> www.helios.co.uk

HOMEOPATHY IN REAL LIFE

The following is a compilation of true stories from acquaintances, friends, and family members who have used homeopathy successfully. The names and some of the details in all of the stories have been changed in order to protect the identity of those involved.

These stories are not a substitute for medical advice, and I don't agree with the choices of every person in these stories. The intention here is to show the power of a well chosen remedy. If you're having a medical emergency, please seek medical attention.

All of the people in these stories followed up with their healthcare practitioners, and were given a clean bill of health.

PINCHED FINGERS

Several years ago, Regina decided to upgrade to a minivan. Her son was 3 at the time, and he insisted on learning to close the sliding door by himself. Although it slid nicely, it was heavy for little guy, and it always took him multiple tries to close it.

One day, Regina was late for an appointment. She figured it would be easier to deal with the objections of her 3 year old, than to be late to the dentist. She reached around from the front seat to close the door, just as her son was using all of his strength to try to close it. Her 3 year old was successful, and the door slammed shut on Regina's fingers.

She quickly pried the door open as pain shot through her fingers. They didn't seem to be broken, but they sure felt like it. She raced back inside for her homeopathy kit. She had just read an article about *hypericum*; one of the best remedies for injuries to nerve rich areas like fingers and toes. A few minutes after taking a dose of *hypericum*, she started to feel the shooting pain diminish and could bend her fingers again. A few minutes after that, the pain returned. She took another dose. It worked again and she was finally on her way to the dentist. After her son got the van door closed, of course.

ANXIETY & HEAT STROKE

Bryan was an anxious teen with above average intelligence, and he had a major fear of water. Much to his dismay, his family decided to spend the day on a beach near his house. Bryan wore his normal clothing, because he had no plans to leave his beach chair and join his family in the water. He had brought a stack of books, and he was going to finish them all that day. His dad had other plans, and he brought his newly purchased homeopathic remedy kit to combat Bryan's anxiety.

When they reached the beach, the sight of the water made Bryan feel dazed and a little shaky. His dad looked those symptoms up in his homeopathy book, recognized that Bryan needed the remedy *aconite,* and gave him a dose. Within about 15 minutes, Bryan started to relax. He began to notice how much fun the others were having in the water. About 30 minutes after the aconite, Bryan inched over to the water and put his toes in. Finally, deciding to join them, he took off his shirt and slowly began to wade into the water.

Bryan played all day with his family, and had such a great time that he forgot to apply sunscreen. On the way home Bryan began to notice his sunburn, but didn't complain much because he was so exhausted. As soon as they arrived home, he quickly fell into bed; only taking the time to ask his mom for another blanket because he felt so cold.

A short while later, Bryan woke up with extreme nausea and a funny feeling in his chest. He ran to the bathroom and immediately began vomiting and having diarrhea. His face was a bright red, he had a high fever, and his heart was racing. His parents were worried he was having a heat stroke, and they began to prepare for a trip to the emergency room. Bryan's dad remembered reading in his homeopathy book that Belladonna was for intense heat stroke. He gave him a dose on the way to the hospital, hoping it would buy them some time to get there. Within 5 minutes, the vomiting, diarrhea, fever, and heart rate had all normalized. His parents were surprised at how quickly it had worked, and grateful they had decided to invest in a remedy kit.

PLANTAR FASCIITIS

Jesse had noticed a pain in her left foot off and on for a while. It was worse in the morning and after she had been sitting for an extended period of time. For the first few months it wasn't really bothersome, so she didn't pay too much attention to it.

One morning, Jesse woke up feeling fine, but as soon as she stepped foot on the floor she screeched in pain and leaped back into bed. She couldn't put any weight on her left foot, and ended up calling in sick to work that day while she tried to figure out what to do.

After a visit to the urgent care center, she was diagnosed with plantar fasciitis. The doctor encouraged her to rest as much as possible, use ice or heat, and look into physical therapy. Jesse had a friend who was into natural health, so she gave her a call. Her friend recommended looking into homeopathy, because it had worked quickly on an injury she had gotten last year. Jesse's friend told her to list out her symptoms, and try to match them to a list of plantar fasciitis remedies she found online.

After a quick search, Jesse found two remedies that seemed like a good match: *graphites* and *zincum metallicum*. They had many crossover symptoms such as cold sweaty feet, swelling, and pain that gets worse with pressure, but there was one peculiar symptom of *zincum metallicum* that stood out to her: nervous fidgety movement of the feet. Jesse remembered she'd had that symptom for quite awhile. She took a few doses of the remedy *zincum metallicum* throughout that week, had a slight improvement with each dose, and was significantly better by the weekend.

Note: most homeopaths would view this as a chronic issue, and would recommend being seen by a homeopathic practitioner.

BURNS

Amy was in a hurry to get dinner on the table and pulled out the pan for spaghetti. As she was putting the pan full of water on the stove, she heard a crash. When she turned around to see what had happened, she touched her arm on the hot stove.

Luckily, the noise was just her toddler overturning his toy bin on the tile floor, but she noticed her arm was beginning to sting. She ran some cold water over it, and started the process of making the sauce for the spaghetti.

While the sauce simmered, she returned to the noodles that now needed to be drained. As she poured the hot water into the sink, the steam from the hot water burned her other arm. She ran cold water over both burns, and finished making dinner. As she got everyone to the table and sat down to eat, she realized both burns were really starting to hurt.

Amy grabbed her homeopathy kit and took a dose of *cantharis*, the most common burn remedy. A few minutes later, she noticed the pain was completely gone from her first burn, but the second burn was feeling much worse. She decided to try another dose of *cantharis*. It still didn't do anything for her second burn, so she grabbed her homeopathy book and turned to the section on burns. She read that the remedy for steam burns with stinging pain is often u*rtica urens*. Luckily, she also had that remedy, and a few minutes after trying it she was pain free.

DEEP WOUND

Andrew was a roofer, and often worked with sharp and dangerous tools. Occasionally, he injured himself. This time, he pulled out his box cutter knife and went to cut through a package of shingles. His knife slipped, and he ended up with a large cut in his leg. Andrew did not have health insurance, and he refused to make the expensive visit to the emergency room; ignoring the advice of his friends and family.

Andrew had a friend that was familiar with first aid and homeopathy. By the time his friend arrived, the wound had stopped bleeding, but there was a large gaping hole. His friend soaked it in a tub of antibacterial wound cleaner mixed with warm water, and started with a few doses of *arnica* because it's a common remedy for injuries.

When that didn't seem to help, he switched to h*ypericum*, because the pain was radiating up and down Andrew's leg. The *hypericum* took care of the pain, he bandaged Andrew up, and sent him home with the remedy *calendula* to help prevent infection and promote healing. A few days later,

Andrew followed up with his doctor. They were both surprised at how quickly the wound was healing.

SEASONAL ALLERGIES

Ben and James were father and son with a lot in common, including seasonal allergies. Every spring, Ben would start to feel the drippy nose, sneezing, runny eyes, and itchy throat. Although James also had hay fever, he experienced completely different symptoms. He struggled with a runny nose, itchy, burning eyes, and a huge desire to rub them.

Both preferred to treat their symptoms naturally before using medications. They decided to look up the most common remedies for seasonal allergies and match their symptoms to a homeopathic remedy. Ben matched the remedy *allium cepa*, which is for a burning dripping nose. James matched the remedy *euphrasia*, which is for allergies that affect the eyes. After a few doses, they both experienced complete relief, and they both started to enjoy springtime again.

REFLUX AND INDIGESTION

For years, Sheryl has needed a dose or two a day of antacid medicine. The medication would always help for a little while, but she would always need another dose. She tried changing her diet and even tried some natural herbs for digestion, but she could never get it completely under control.

One day, when her friend was visiting, Sheryl felt the need to reach for her antacid. Her friend handed her a bottle she had in the bottom of her purse instead. It was labeled cell salt #10 *natrum sulph*. She tried a dose, and her indigestion subsided. Impressed, she ordered her own bottle and saw similar results every time. After a few months of use, she needed it less and less. Eventually she forgot that she even struggled with acid reflux.

SCRATCHED CORNEA

Pete was around seven years old when he started helping his dad with woodworking. It was late fall when they decided to take on their biggest project yet: a play table for Pete's room. After finishing the table structure, they needed to do some sanding.

As Pete's dad turned on the sander and began to move it across the table, a gust of wind blew a huge cloud of sawdust straight into Pete's face. He had no time to blink and several pieces went into his eye. Pete began rubbing his eye, and after a few minutes Pete's eye was bright red and he was in a large amount of pain. Pete's dad helped him rinse his eye in the shower, but it made no difference.

Pete's parents decided to take him into a local urgent care center. The doctor looked in his eye and did not see any debris. Next, she put some drops in his eye to check for scratches. It was obvious that Pete had scratched his cornea. The doctor said that it would take several weeks for it to heal.

Pete was very fearful and crying most of the visit. He was scared he would lose his vision and was trembling. Pete's mom called her homeopath, who helped walk her through the process of finding a remedy. Since *aconite* is considered one of the best remedies for the eyes. they started there.

After one dose of *aconite*, Pete was starting to feel better. The pain in his eye was diminishing, and so was his fear. About an hour later, Pete was starting to get nervous again. His mother gave Pete another dose of *aconite,* and within a few minutes he returned to his normal self. He no longer complained of pain in his eye and the redness was gone. They repeated *aconite* a few times over the next few days, until Pete's symptoms stopped returning.

GRIEF

Amy had a cat named Francis that she adored. Every morning, the cat would wait outside her door for her to wake up, and they would spend the morning together. Amy knew Francis was not feeling well when she didn't meet her for their normal morning routine. Amy took the day off from work, and took Francis to the vet. It was bad news: Francis was very ill and needed to be put down.

She was devastated, but knew it was the right thing to do. On the way home from the vet, Amy couldn't stop crying. Her husband reminded her that grieving was normal, especially after the loss of a pet she had been close to for so long.

Several weeks later, Amy was still struggling. She became withdrawn, and cried every day in her car before heading into work. Her appetite was gone, and she often ended her sentences with a sigh. Her husband was worried and reached out to their homeopath for help. The homeopath suggested the remedy *ignatia*, because it seemed to fit Amy's symptoms well.

Amy took a dose, and for the first time in weeks she felt the depression lift. She was able to talk about Francis without bursting into tears. After a few doses of *ignatia* over the next few days, Amy started talking through her grief in a healthy way, and she finally felt like life was getting back to normal. She even started talking about the future and the possibility of getting another cat some day.

HOMEOPATHIC FIRST AID REMEDIES

CUTS/SCRAPES/BLEEDING:

Arnica, Hypericum, Ledum, Calendula, Phosphorus, Belladonna

INJURIES/SPRAINS/STRAINS:

Arnica, Ruta, Rhus Tox, Bryonia

HEAT EXHAUSTION/HEAT STROKE:

Belladonna, Gloinine

SUNBURN:

Arnica, Cantharis, Causticum, Urtica

HEADACHES:

Natrum Muriaticum, Belladonna, Bryonia, Gelsemium, Sanguinaria, Spigelia, Iris

FOOD POISONING:

Arsenicum, Ipecac, Nux Vomica, Podophyllum, Pulsatilla, Veratrum, Urtica,

DIARRHEA:

Aloe, Arsenicum, Podophyllum, Sulphur, Veratrum

ALLERGIC REACTION:

Apis, Allium Cepa, Arsenicum, Rhus Tox, Urtica

FEVER:

Belladonna, Aconite, China, Ferrum Phos

FEAR OF FLYING:

Aconite, Argentum, Arsenicum, Calc Carb

MOTION SICKNESS:

Cocculus, Sepia, Tabacum, Petroleum

SHOCK/FRIGHT:

Aconite, Arnica, Carbo Veg, China, Veratrum

HEAD INJURY:

Arnica, Hypericum, Nat Sulph

INDIGESTION/STOMACH PAIN:

Nat Phos #10, Bryonia, Colocynthis, Mag Phos, Lycopodium, Nux Vomica, Pulsatilla

INSECT BITES/STINGS:

Apis, Caladium, Carbolicum acidum, Ledum, Vespa

TOOTHACHE:

Chamomila, Coffea, Hepar Sulph, Mercurius, Plantago

STAGE FRIGHT:

Lycopodium, Gelsemium, Argentum

INSOMNIA:

Coffea, Aconite, Arsenicum, Chamomila, Gelsemium, Ignatia, Nux Vomica

GRIEF:

Natrum Muriaticum, Ignatia, Phosphoric acid

COLD/FLU:

Ferrum Phos, Aconite, Influenzinum, Oscillococcinum, Belladonna, Pulsatilla, Apis Mellifica, Gelsemium, Bryonia, Rhus Tox

COUGH:

Bryonia, Drosera, Hepar Sulph, Ipecac, Phosphorus, Pulsatilla, Rumex, Spongia, Coccus Cacti

DISCLAIMER

I am not a certified homeopath or a licensed health care practitioner. I'm a mom who has struggled to walk her family through a variety of health issues, and has used homeopathy as part of our journey. The goal of this book is not to debate the effectiveness or validity of homeopathy, and the book does not provide a detailed explanation of how it works. There are other resources that address these issues. I simply wish to share what I've learned in an easy to read introduction to homeopathy.

This book is not a substitute for any medical treatment or the advice of a licensed physician. It is not intended to diagnose, treat, or cure any disease or ailment. If you are experiencing a medical emergency, please seek emergency medical treatment immediately.

The books and websites I discuss in this book are the ones I use the most. I have no affiliation with any of these resources, and I did not receive any compensation for mentioning these in this book.

Made in United States
Troutdale, OR
11/23/2024

25190783R00046